How to Lose Your Virginity without Pain

Beginners Guide on Building a Positive Attitude toward Sex, Educating Yourself about Your Body and Enjoying Yourself during Sex

Wendy Chad

How to Lose Your Virginity without Pain

First Edition: 2024

Printed in United States of America

Distributed by Amazon.com, Inc.

Wendy Chad

Dedication

To everyone embarking on the journey of self-discovery and intimacy, may this guide empower you with confidence, knowledge, and joy as you explore the beautiful realm of sexuality.

Table of Contents

Introduction

The journey towards sexual intimacy is a deeply personal and often complex path. Losing your virginity is a significant milestone that can be accompanied by a mixture of excitement, curiosity, and apprehension. "How to Lose Your Virginity without Pain: Beginners Guide on Building a Positive Attitude toward Sex, Educating Yourself about Your Body and Enjoying Yourself during Sex" is designed to be your comprehensive guide, helping you navigate this important life event with confidence, knowledge, and ease.

Embracing a Positive Attitude towards Sex

One of the foundational elements of a healthy sexual experience is a positive attitude towards sex.

How to Lose Your Virginity without Pain

Unfortunately, societal stigmas, cultural expectations, and personal anxieties can cloud our perceptions and create unnecessary pressure. This book begins by addressing the importance of building a positive and healthy outlook on sex. By fostering a mindset that embraces sex as a natural, enjoyable, and intimate act, you can eliminate much of the fear and anxiety associated with losing your virginity. We'll explore practical strategies for cultivating this positive attitude, ensuring you are mentally and emotionally prepared for this new chapter.

The Importance of Readiness

Sex is a significant and intimate act that should be approached with care and consideration. Ensuring that you are truly ready—emotionally, mentally, and physically—is crucial. This book will guide you through the signs of readiness, helping you to recognize and honor your own boundaries and desires.

Wendy Chad

Understanding and respecting your own readiness can transform your first sexual experience from one of apprehension to one of mutual respect and pleasure.

Communicating with Your Partner

Effective communication is the cornerstone of a positive sexual experience. Discussing your fears, expectations, and boundaries with your partner before, during, and after sex can create a foundation of trust and mutual respect. This book offers practical advice on how to initiate these important conversations, fostering an environment where both partners feel comfortable, understood, and valued. By establishing open lines of communication, you can navigate any uncertainties together and ensure that the experience is consensual and enjoyable for both parties.

Educating Yourself about Your Body

Knowledge is empowering, especially when it comes to understanding your own body. This book provides a detailed exploration of female anatomy, sexual response cycles, and the mechanics of intercourse. By educating yourself about your body and how sex works, you can approach your first sexual experience with greater confidence and less fear. Topics such as discovering your hymen, identifying the angle of your vagina, and locating your clitoris are discussed in detail, empowering you with the knowledge needed to fully understand and enjoy your body.

Creating a Comfortable and Relaxing Environment

The environment in which you choose to have sex for the first time can greatly influence your experience. This book offers practical tips on how to create a stress-free, comfortable, and intimate setting. From choosing the right location and setting a relaxing mood to ensuring privacy and reducing distractions, these guidelines will help you create an atmosphere that enhances comfort and pleasure. A thoughtful environment can alleviate anxiety and promote relaxation, making the experience more enjoyable and less intimidating.

Ensuring Safety and Comfort

Safety and comfort are paramount in any sexual experience, but they are especially important when losing your virginity. This book emphasizes the importance of using protection, applying lubricant, and taking your time. These steps are not only crucial for physical comfort but also for emotional well-being. By prioritizing safety and comfort, you can prevent physical discomfort and emotional distress, allowing you to focus on the pleasurable and intimate aspects of the experience.

Enjoying the Experience

Ultimately, the goal of this book is to help you enjoy your first sexual experience. We'll explore strategies for relaxation, techniques for enhancing pleasure, and the importance of aftercare. By learning how to communicate your needs, set a comfortable pace, and engage in mutual care after the act, you can ensure that your first experience is positive, pleasurable, and memorable. Enjoying the experience means being present, letting go of anxieties, and focusing on the connection and pleasure shared with your partner.

A Journey of Self-Discovery

Losing your virginity is more than just a physical act; it's a journey of self-discovery and personal growth. This book encourages you to view this milestone as an opportunity to learn about yourself, your desires, and your boundaries. Each step of the journey—from building a positive attitude to educating yourself about your body and enjoying the experience—contributes to a deeper understanding of your own sexuality.

Moving Forward with Confidence

As you embark on this journey, remember that there is no one "right" way to lose your virginity. What matters most is that you feel ready, comfortable, and informed. This book is here to guide you every step of the way, providing you with the knowledge and tools needed to ensure a positive and pain-free experience. Embrace this journey with confidence, knowing that you have the support and information needed to make it a fulfilling and enjoyable experience.

In conclusion, "How to Lose Your Virginity without Pain: Beginners Guide on Building a Positive Attitude toward Sex, Educating Yourself about Your Body and Enjoying Yourself during Sex" is your comprehensive resource for navigating this important life event. By building a positive attitude, educating yourself, and creating a comfortable environment, you can ensure that your first sexual experience is one of pleasure, intimacy, and mutual respect.

Part 1: Building a Positive Attitude

How to Lose Your Virginity without Pain

Embarking on the journey to lose your virginity is a significant milestone in your sexual development, and it's essential to approach it with a positive attitude. Cultivating a healthy mindset towards sex involves several key steps, each designed to empower you and enhance your overall sexual experience.

Assess Your Readiness

Understanding Emotional and Mental Readiness: Before engaging in sexual activity, it's crucial to assess your emotional and mental readiness. Consider your feelings towards sex, your level of comfort with your partner, and any concerns or fears you may have. Being emotionally and mentally prepared ensures that you approach sex with confidence and clarity.

Reflecting on Personal Values and Desires: Take time to reflect on your personal values and desires regarding sex. Consider what sex means to you, what you hope to gain from the experience, and whether it aligns with your values and beliefs. Understanding your motivations for wanting to lose your virginity can help you make informed decisions and approach the experience with intention.

Exploring Boundaries and Preferences: Establish clear boundaries and preferences for yourself before engaging in sexual activity. Communicate these boundaries to your partner and ensure that they are respected throughout the experience. Knowing your limits and preferences can help you feel more comfortable and in control during intimate moments.

Communicate with Your Partner

Open and Honest Communication: Effective communication with your partner is essential for a positive sexual experience. Discuss your thoughts, feelings, and expectations regarding sex openly and honestly. Encourage your partner to do the same and create a safe space for open dialogue and mutual understanding.

Expressing Concerns and Boundaries: Take the opportunity to express any concerns or boundaries you may have with your partner. Be clear and assertive about what you are comfortable with and what you are not. Establishing clear communication around boundaries ensures that both you and your partner feel respected and supported throughout the experience.

Creating Mutual Understanding: Foster mutual understanding and respect with your partner by actively listening to their needs and desires. Seek to understand their perspective and be willing to compromise and accommodate each other's preferences. Building a foundation of mutual trust and respect is essential for a positive and fulfilling sexual relationship.

Seeking Guidance from Trusted Adults

Identifying Trusted Adults: Identify trusted adults in your life whom you can turn to for guidance and support regarding sex. This may include parents, guardians, older siblings, or trusted mentors. Choose individuals who you feel comfortable confiding in and who can provide you with accurate information and guidance.

Initiating Open Discussions: Initiate open and honest discussions with trusted adults about sex and sexuality. Approach these conversations with curiosity and a willingness to learn. Ask questions, seek advice, and share your thoughts and concerns openly. Trusted adults can offer valuable insights and support as you navigate your sexual journey.

Accessing Reliable Resources: Seek out reliable resources and educational materials on sex and sexual health. Books, websites, and educational programs can provide valuable information on topics such as consent, contraception, STI prevention, and sexual pleasure. Educating yourself with accurate and up-to-date information empowers you to make informed decisions about your sexual health and well-being.

Part 2: Educating Yourself about Your Body

How to Lose Your Virginity without Pain

Understanding your body and its functions is a crucial step towards having a positive and enjoyable first sexual experience. This chapter will guide you through the essential aspects of educating yourself about your body, helping you build confidence and awareness. By learning about how sex works, discovering your hymen, identifying the angle of your vagina, and locating your clitoris, you'll be well-prepared to embark on this intimate journey.

Learn About How Sex Works

The Basics of Sexual Intercourse: Sexual intercourse, or penetrative sex, involves the insertion of the penis into the vagina. This act can vary in depth, speed, and rhythm, depending on the preferences of both partners. Understanding the mechanics of sex can help demystify the experience and reduce any anxiety you might have.

The Role of Arousal and Lubrication: Arousal plays a significant role in preparing your body for sex. When you're aroused, your body produces natural lubrication, which reduces friction and makes penetration more comfortable. Engaging in foreplay, such as kissing, touching, and oral sex, can help increase arousal and lubrication.

The Importance of Communication: Clear communication with your partner about what feels good and what doesn't is essential. Discussing your likes, dislikes, and any concerns before and during sex can lead to a more enjoyable and comfortable experience. Don't be afraid to speak up and guide your partner.

Discover Your Hymen

What is the Hymen? The hymen is a thin membrane that partially covers the vaginal opening. It varies greatly in shape, size, and thickness from person to person. Contrary to popular belief, the hymen doesn't "break" during sex; it can stretch or tear, which might cause some discomfort or light bleeding.

Understanding Hymen Variability: The state of the hymen can differ significantly among individuals. Some women have very little hymenal tissue, while others have more. Physical activities like sports or using tampons can also cause the hymen to stretch or tear, which is perfectly normal.

Addressing Hymen Myths: There are many myths surrounding the hymen, such as the idea that it should be intact before sex. Educating yourself about the hymen helps dispel these myths and reduces unnecessary anxiety. Remember, the presence or condition of the hymen is not an indicator of virginity or sexual activity.

Identify the Angle of Your Vagina

Anatomy of the Vagina: The vagina is a muscular canal that leads from the vaginal opening to the cervix. It has a natural angle that can vary among individuals. Understanding your vaginal anatomy can help you and your partner find comfortable and pleasurable positions during sex.

Exploring with a Mirror: Using a mirror to look at your vaginal area can help you become familiar with your anatomy. Gently exploring with clean fingers can also help you understand the angle and depth of your vagina, which can be beneficial when guiding your partner during penetration.

Experimenting with Positions: Different sexual positions can affect the angle of penetration.

How to Lose Your Virginity without Pain

Experimenting with various positions, such as missionary, spooning, or woman on top, can help you find the angles that feel most comfortable and pleasurable for you.

Locate Your Clitoris

Understanding the Clitoris: The clitoris is a highly sensitive organ located at the top of the vulva, just above the vaginal opening. It is composed of a glans (the visible part), a body, and internal roots that extend into the pelvis. The clitoris is primarily responsible for sexual pleasure and arousal in women.

Exploring Your Clitoris: Take time to explore your clitoris using your fingers. Gentle rubbing, tapping, or circular motions can help you discover what feels best. Using lubrication can enhance the experience and prevent discomfort.

Incorporating Clitoral Stimulation: During sex, incorporating clitoral stimulation can enhance pleasure and increase the likelihood of orgasm. You can stimulate your clitoris with your fingers, a vibrator, or ask your partner to do so. Communicate your needs and preferences to your partner to ensure a satisfying experience.

Putting It All Together

Combining Knowledge and Practice: Now that you have a better understanding of your body, it's time to put this knowledge into practice. Use what you've learned about the mechanics of sex, your hymen, vaginal angle, and clitoris to guide your sexual experiences.

Engaging in Self-Exploration: Masturbation is a healthy and natural way to explore your body and discover what feels good. It can help you become more comfortable with your anatomy and increase your sexual confidence.

Educating Your Partner: Sharing your knowledge with your partner can improve your sexual experiences together. Teaching them about your body

How to Lose Your Virginity without Pain

and what you enjoy can enhance intimacy and mutual satisfaction.

Overcoming Challenges

Dealing with Anxiety: It's normal to feel anxious about your first sexual experience. Practice deep breathing, mindfulness, or other relaxation techniques to help calm your nerves. Remember, sex is a learning experience, and it's okay to take things slow.

Addressing Discomfort: If you experience discomfort during sex, communicate with your partner and adjust your approach. Trying different positions, using more lubrication, or taking breaks can help alleviate discomfort.

Seeking Professional Advice: If you have concerns or experience persistent pain during sex, consider consulting a healthcare professional. They can provide guidance, address any medical issues, and

How to Lose Your Virginity without Pain

offer advice on how to make sex more comfortable and enjoyable.

By taking the time to educate yourself about your body and understanding how sex works, you can approach your first sexual experience with confidence and clarity. This knowledge will not only help you feel more comfortable but also empower you to have a positive and enjoyable experience.

Part 3: Enjoying Yourself during Sex

How to Lose Your Virginity without Pain

Losing your virginity is a significant milestone, and ensuring that the experience is pleasurable and enjoyable is paramount. This chapter will guide you through essential steps to create a positive and memorable first sexual encounter. By picking a stress-free location, setting a relaxing mood, getting consent, using protection, applying lubricant, taking your time, communicating your needs, and doing some aftercare, you can maximize your enjoyment and minimize any potential discomfort or anxiety.

Pick a Stress-Free Location

Choose a Comfortable Space: The location of your first sexual experience plays a crucial role in ensuring comfort and relaxation. Select a space where you feel safe and at ease. This could be your bedroom or any place that is familiar and private.

Minimize Interruptions: To fully enjoy the moment, it's important to minimize any potential interruptions. Make sure you are in a place where you won't be disturbed by roommates, family members, or other distractions. Lock the door if necessary to ensure privacy.

Create a Clean Environment: A clean and tidy environment can significantly impact your mood. Take a few minutes to clean the space, change the bed sheets, and remove any clutter. This helps create a more inviting and relaxing atmosphere.

Control the Temperature: Ensure that the room is at a comfortable temperature. Being too hot or too cold can be distracting and uncomfortable. Adjust the thermostat, use fans, or add blankets as needed to create a cozy environment.

Personalize the Space: Add personal touches to the room to make it feel more intimate. This could include adding some pillows, a favorite blanket, or any other items that make you feel comfortable and relaxed.

Set a Relaxing Mood

Lighting: Soft, dim lighting can help create a calming and intimate ambiance. Use lamps, fairy lights, or candles to achieve a warm glow. Avoid harsh, bright lights that can be unsettling.

Scent: Pleasant scents can enhance the mood and make the experience more enjoyable. Consider using scented candles, incense, or essential oils like lavender or vanilla, which have calming properties.

Sound: Music can play a powerful role in setting the mood. Create a playlist of your favorite songs that are soothing and sensual. The right music can help both of you relax and get into the moment.

Eliminate Distractions: Turn off any potential distractions, such as your phone or television. Focus on creating an environment where you can both fully immerse yourselves in the experience without interruptions.

Comfortable Seating or Bedding: Make sure that the bed or seating arrangement is comfortable. Adding extra pillows or a soft blanket can make a significant difference in how comfortable and relaxed you feel.

Get Consent

Discuss Boundaries: Before engaging in any sexual activity, have an open and honest conversation with your partner about boundaries and limits. Knowing each other's comfort zones can prevent misunderstandings and ensure a respectful experience.

Mutual Agreement: Consent should be enthusiastic and mutual. Both partners should feel equally willing and excited about the experience. If either of you feels unsure or pressured, it's important to pause and discuss your feelings.

Ongoing Consent: Consent isn't a one-time check. Continuously check in with each other throughout the experience to ensure that both of you are comfortable and willing to proceed. This can be as simple as asking, "Is this okay?" or "Do you like this?"

Respecting Decisions: If either partner decides to stop at any point, that decision should be respected without question. Comfort and safety should always come first.

Clear Communication: Use clear and direct communication to express your desires and boundaries. This helps prevent any misunderstandings and ensures that both partners are on the same page.

Use Protection

Types of Protection: Using protection is crucial to prevent sexually transmitted infections (STIs) and unwanted pregnancies. Condoms are the most common form of protection and are readily available.

Correct Usage: Ensure that you know how to correctly use condoms. Check the expiration date, open the package carefully, and follow the instructions for application. This ensures maximum effectiveness.

Have Protection Ready: Keep protection within easy reach so you don't have to interrupt the moment to find it. Being prepared helps maintain the flow of the experience.

Discuss Protection Preferences: Have a conversation with your partner about your preferred methods of protection. Agree on what you will use before you begin to avoid any last-minute confusion or discomfort.

Double-Check: Double-check that the condom is on properly and hasn't broken during use. If you're unsure, take a moment to check and replace it if necessary.

Apply Lubricant

Why Lubrication Matters: Lubrication reduces friction, making penetration smoother and more comfortable. This is especially important if you're nervous or if it's your first time, as anxiety can reduce natural lubrication.

Types of Lubricants: There are various types of lubricants available, including water-based, silicone-based, and oil-based. Water-based lubricants are the most versatile and safe to use with condoms.

Application: Apply a generous amount of lubricant to the condom and to yourself before penetration. Don't be afraid to reapply as needed to maintain comfort.

Avoid Irritants: Choose a lubricant that is free from irritants like glycerin or parabens, especially if you have sensitive skin. Opt for products specifically designed for sexual use.

Communicate Needs: If you feel any discomfort or dryness during sex, don't hesitate to ask your partner to pause so you can apply more lubricant. Communication ensures that both partners remain comfortable and enjoy the experience.

Take Your Time

Pace Yourselves: There's no need to rush. Take your time to explore each other's bodies and enjoy the journey. Rushing can lead to discomfort and anxiety, while a slower pace allows for more pleasure and connection.

Foreplay: Engaging in ample foreplay helps increase arousal and natural lubrication. Kissing, touching, oral sex, and other intimate activities can enhance your experience and build anticipation.

Listen to Your Body: Pay attention to your body's signals. If something feels uncomfortable or painful, slow down or try a different approach. Your comfort and pleasure are paramount.

Explore Together: Use this time to explore what feels good for both of you. Experiment with different touches, pressures, and rhythms. This exploration can deepen your connection and increase mutual satisfaction.

Build Trust: Taking your time helps build trust and intimacy between partners. Trust is essential for a positive sexual experience, especially when it's your first time.

Communicate Your Needs

Verbal Communication: Clearly express what you like and don't like during sex. Saying things like "That feels good" or "Can you try this?" helps guide your partner and enhances your experience.

Non-Verbal Cues: Pay attention to non-verbal cues from your partner. Moans, gasps, and body language can provide important feedback about what feels good and what doesn't.

Feedback Loop: Create a feedback loop where both partners feel comfortable giving and receiving feedback. This open communication fosters a more pleasurable and satisfying experience.

Adjusting Techniques: Be willing to adjust techniques based on feedback. What works for one person might not work for another, so being adaptable is key to mutual pleasure.

Respect and Patience: Communicate with respect and patience. Remember that both partners are learning and exploring together, so a kind and patient approach helps maintain a positive atmosphere.

Do Some Aftercare

Physical Comfort: Aftercare involves tending to each other's physical comfort after sex. This could include cuddling, holding each other, or sharing a shower together. Physical closeness helps reinforce the bond you've created.

Emotional Check-In: Check in with each other emotionally. Discuss how you felt about the experience, what you enjoyed, and any concerns you might have. This open dialogue strengthens your emotional connection.

Hydration and Hygiene: Drinking water and attending to personal hygiene after sex is important. Use this time to clean up and ensure that both partners feel refreshed and comfortable.

Affirmations and Reassurance: Offer affirmations and reassurance to each other. Expressing love, appreciation, and satisfaction reinforces positive feelings and boosts confidence.

Reflect and Learn: Reflect on the experience and discuss what you've learned. This helps you both understand each other's needs and preferences better, leading to more fulfilling experiences in the future.

By following these steps, you can create a positive and enjoyable sexual experience. Remember, the key to enjoying yourself during sex is to focus on comfort, communication, and mutual respect. Take your time, be present in the moment, and prioritize your and your partner's pleasure and well-being. This approach will help ensure that your first time is a memorable and positive experience.

Conclusion

Embarking on the journey of losing your virginity is a significant and personal milestone. It's a moment that marks a new chapter in your life, one filled with excitement, curiosity, and perhaps a bit of anxiety. This book, "How to Lose Your Virginity without Pain: Beginners Guide on Building a Positive Attitude toward Sex, Educating Yourself about Your Body and Enjoying Yourself during Sex," has aimed to provide you with comprehensive guidance to ensure that this experience is positive, empowering, and as pain-free as possible.

Reflecting on Your Readiness

Throughout the chapters, we've emphasized the importance of being ready. Readiness is not just about physical preparedness but also emotional and mental readiness. Understanding and respecting your own boundaries and desires is crucial. By ensuring that you are truly ready, you can approach the experience with confidence and excitement rather than fear and hesitation. Remember, there's no rush. Taking the time to ensure you're ready can make a significant difference in your overall experience.

Communicating with Your Partner

Communication is the cornerstone of a healthy and enjoyable sexual experience. We've discussed the importance of open, honest, and ongoing communication with your partner. By discussing your fears, expectations, and boundaries beforehand, you can build a foundation of trust and mutual respect. This dialogue should continue during and after the experience to ensure that both partners feel comfortable and satisfied. Effective communication can transform a potentially awkward experience into one of deep connection and mutual pleasure.

Seeking Guidance and Support

Having a trusted adult or confidant to talk to can provide invaluable support and perspective. This person can offer advice, answer questions, and help you navigate any uncertainties you may have. Knowing that you have someone to turn to can alleviate some of the pressure and make the experience feel less isolating. Remember, seeking guidance is a sign of strength and wisdom, not weakness.

Educating Yourself about Your Body

Knowledge is power, especially when it comes to understanding your own body. We've covered the importance of educating yourself about how sex works, discovering your hymen, identifying the angle of your vagina, and locating your clitoris. This self-awareness empowers you to take control of your sexual experiences and communicate your needs more effectively. By understanding your body, you can enhance your pleasure and reduce any potential discomfort.

Creating a Positive and Relaxing Environment

The environment in which you have sex can significantly impact your experience. We've discussed how to choose a stress-free location, set a relaxing mood, and create an atmosphere that promotes comfort and intimacy. By taking control of these factors, you can create a space where you feel safe, relaxed, and ready to enjoy the moment. The right environment can help reduce anxiety and make the experience more pleasurable.

Ensuring Safety and Comfort

Safety and comfort are paramount. Using protection, applying lubricant, and taking your time are all essential steps to ensure that your first experience is safe and enjoyable. These measures help prevent physical discomfort and emotional distress. By prioritizing safety and comfort, you can focus on the positive aspects of the experience and fully enjoy the moment.

Enjoying the Experience

The ultimate goal of this guide is to help you enjoy your first sexual experience. We've provided tips on how to relax, take your time, communicate your needs, and engage in aftercare. By following these steps, you can create a positive, pleasurable, and memorable experience. Enjoying the experience means being present in the moment, letting go of fears, and focusing on the pleasure and connection with your partner.

Reflecting on the Journey

As you conclude this book, take a moment to reflect on the journey you've undertaken. From building a positive attitude to educating yourself about your body and learning how to enjoy sex, you've equipped yourself with the knowledge and tools needed for a positive experience. This journey is ongoing, and each experience will provide new insights and opportunities for growth.

Moving Forward

Remember, losing your virginity is just the beginning of your sexual journey. Each experience will be unique, and it's important to continue learning and growing. Maintain open communication with your partner, keep educating yourself about your body, and prioritize your own comfort and pleasure. By doing so, you will continue to build positive and fulfilling sexual experiences.

Final Thoughts

In closing, losing your virginity is a deeply personal and significant experience. By following the guidance provided in this book, you can approach this milestone with confidence, knowledge, and a positive attitude. Remember, the most important aspect of any sexual experience is mutual respect and enjoyment. Take your time, communicate openly, and prioritize your own well-being. Here's to a positive, empowering, and pain-free journey into your sexual life.